How I Finally Got Rid Of Angular Cheilitis Once and For All!
Cracked Mouth Corners No More

HEATHER KALE

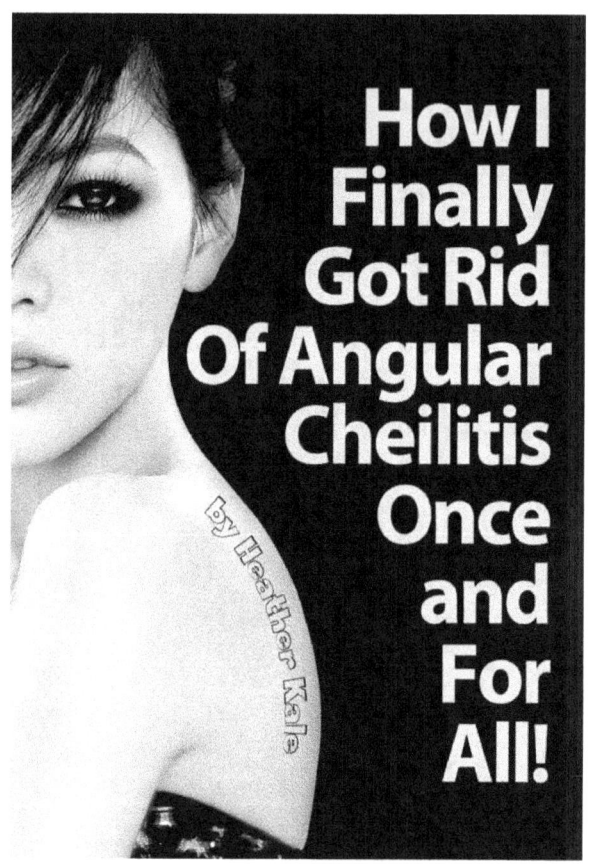

How I Finally

GOT RID OF MY

ANGULAR CHEILITIS

ISBN-13: 978-1503374850

ISBN-10: 1503374858

All Rights Reserved 2014

HEATHER KALE

ONCE AND FOR ALL

Contents

1 Introduction

When you see something advertised on TV, you know that you are watching an actor or actress who has been paid to endorse a product or tell you about the cure that they are pitching. Because of that, many people take personal endorsements with a grain of salt because it is easy for anybody to claim that something works when they do not know. I wrote this book because I wanted to have a very real, down to earth personal account of my experience and my struggle with Angular Cheilitis including how I was able to cure it, ending years and years of frustration.

I know there are others that have struggled with the same frustration that I have over the failure of most treatments to alleviate or cure their Angular Cheilitis. If something works, then that solution should be shared and that is why I wrote this book.

You see, not every cure has to come along with a product pitch or brand name attached to it. For years, I tried every product out there and found nothing but disappointment. Then I decided that maybe there was another way and that if I fully understood Angular Cheilitis, maybe I could work towards finding a solution that could work for me. I was just relying on what others told me: recommended treatments and solutions I read about online and in forums, but they always fell short.

The answer is yes. Now, when I tell you what it is, you might laugh.

But you are probably reading this because you are an Angular Cheilitis sufferer, so laughing probably hurts. I know this because I suffered for years with it and I am here to tell you that this simple solution will let you laugh again, and do everything that you used to before Angular Cheilitis. Say goodbye to pain and start living life with a smile again!   Sounds like a cheesy commercial I know...

In this case, unusual works.

This cure, however odd, actually worked for me-- and that is why I am here 'speaking' to you, in this book. Other people need to know. I tell anyone I strike up a conversation with—but only if they bring it up—no one likes admitting they get cracked mouth corners on a regular basis.

One of the best things about this is that you will start to feel relief that same day, and your condition will only improve as you continue with the treatment.

Stop waiting for weeks to find relief, you can start to feel better within 24 hours. Can any other cream or medication offer the same? If you are like me, you have already tried an assortment of drugs and creams and found only marginal success.

Not only do they not work very well, but also the regularly used creams and drugs are expensive! When you go from product to product and medicine to medicine and still find no relief it is beyond frustrating. I cannot even tell you how much money I threw at cures and treatments that did not work. By the way, that is exactly why the price of this book is so low: I want you to save money and learn about this simple method—I hope you share this with other sufferers…

Maybe you're thinking 'OK Heather, if the treatments that the experts recommend fail to work, how can you, just a regular person who has suffered from Angular Cheilitis, have the solution?"

Well, I may not be a medical expert but I am somebody who has suffered from Angular

Cheilitis for many years and nothing that I tried ever worked fully. It always came back.

Always, at least until I discovered this amazingly simple cure, which I am about to share with you. My motive is not to sell you expensive and overpriced creams; it is to provide people with a simple yet affordable solution to a problem that I am painfully familiar with.

This solution was actually given to me by somebody else during a casual conversation. I was at a business conference for my previous job. While I was sitting waiting for one of the lectures to start, I started chatting with a woman sitting next to me. I had complimented her on the cute lipstick container on her lap. She was touching up her face (probably because there were tons of handsome men at this event). I had commented on the gorgeous color of her lipstick and when she offered to write down the brand and shade, I declined, pointing to the sides of my mouth--the deep splits were there because of my Angular Cheilitis. Unfortunately I could only wear gobs of lip balm to this event, and this is why sometimes I had to give up wearing foundation too! Otherwise it would 'cake up' in the cracks and look like spackling. Maybe you don't know what spackling is but that's OK—just know that I was always embarrassed whenever I had these flare-ups…

So this gal…she offered me a solution that made me just sit and blink at her.

I did not want her to know that I immediately thought to myself "that will never work and I am not going to try that." I thanked her and pretty much immediately dismissed what she said.

However, I found that later on, my mind just kept going back to what she said and I found myself wondering if something so unusual would actually work.

It does work. It worked for me, and quickly!

I am not passing on knowledge that I have not tried myself. However, instead of just providing a cure, I am also including information about what Angular Cheilitis is and some of the root causes of it. It makes no sense to use the treatment, which will work, only to have your Angular Cheilitis keep coming back. So if you decide to skip over to the 'how to cure' section: after you are done, PLEASE read the rest of this book so you know how to keep it from coming back.

2 Angular Cheilitis – What is it?

Chances are, if you have Angular Cheilitis, you know what it is but it is important to really understand what it is and so this chapter will delve into just what Angular Cheilitis is. You might know that you have it, but not really what it is and what it means to have Angular Cheilitis.

Angular Cheilitis is usually considered to be a type of stomatitis or cheilitis. Often, it is also a type of oral candidiasis because of the lesions that form due to Candida but not all Angular Cheilitis is due to candidiasis. Sometimes it is something that happens rarely, but for many, their Angular Cheilitis is a chronic condition.

When you have Angular Cheilitis, there is an infection of the mouth and lips that presents as deep lines in the corners of the mouth, and inflamed lesions and cuts that appear in the corners of the mouth. These lesions look like small cuts and they hurt, it makes everyday things painful to do and it is embarrassing to have because it is unsightly. Although lips can become chapped, the majority of the problem is situated at the corners of the mouth.

Some Angular Cheilitis sufferers only have it on

one side of their mouth but many, and I was one of these, had it on both sides of the mouth. The corners of the mouth can turn a whitish grey or frightfully red. Skin around the mouth can often be irritated to the point of cracking, in addition to the sores that can develop on the lips and corners of the mouth too.

It is not something that is contagious; you cannot get it from somebody else nor did somebody give it to you.

The sores can often be similar to what you would get from fever blisters or cold sores and thus, many people end up mistreating their Angular Cheilitis because they have misdiagnosed themselves. Cold sore medication is not the way to go and the only way that many people discover that what they have is Angular Cheilitis is because cold sore remedies fail to work and so they seek out their doctor for the answer.

It is not spreadable to another person but it can and will spread easily from one side of your mouth to the other. If you have Angular Cheilitis in one corner of your mouth, you need to be careful how you use your lipstick or chapstick [any lip balm]. If you use the same tube of chapstick on the unaffected corner of your mouth as the infected corner of your mouth, then you will help facilitate the spread of Angular Cheilitis to the other side of your mouth. Just touching the infected side of your mouth with your finger and then touching the other side of your lips can also spread it to the other corner of your mouth.

It often starts with the skin around the mouth turning dry and flaky along with minor redness and irritation that comes along with pain when you try to open your mouth wide.

At this point, most people, me included just think it is from having chapped lips and try to double up on the chapstick, which usually does nothing but spread the problem from one side of your mouth to the other.

As Angular Cheilitis progresses, it becomes painful to open your mouth at all. Blister-like sores will appear in the corner of the mouth and then the corners of the mouth will split, leaving deep, painful open lines that simply will not heal.

Eating anything spicy, acidic or salty causes pain as it hits the open wounds.

I had to immediately change my diet to avoid things that I loved because I knew that it would hurt to eat them. If you have the same deep splits in your mouth that I had, you know exactly what I am talking about. Even if you just have a minor case, you still feel the sting of food hitting the sores and you know that every bite will do the same thing.

Now, I expect you to shake your head and think

that I am nuts when I tell you the cure but let me tell you that I had the same reaction. However, it works. I promise you, it will work, no matter how unusual it sounds!

Now, what makes this cure so different from the usual treatments of steroid creams and anti-fungals? Keep reading to find out!

How I Finally Got Rid Of Angular Cheilitis Once and For All!

3 Using Steroid Creams and Anti-Fungals

Most of the standard solutions to Angular Cheilitis involve using steroid creams and anti-fungals that are topical. I have tried various anti-fungals. I have tried various steroid creams. I have combined the two and yet the Angular Cheilitis never fully would go away. And I have spent tons of dollars on these things for years…

Granted, there are worse and more painful conditions to have than Angular Cheilitis but when nearly every movement of your mouth causes pain and that is combined by how unsightly your mouth looks with Angular Cheilitis, it is not something that you want to live with for very long.

It affects your self-esteem and you become very self-conscious about how your mouth looks. Opening your mouth very wide hurts and it is just overall very frustrating. I used to walk around with my head hanging down, and I'd even wear dark glasses and colour my hair dark. Then I'd powder my entire face with mineral powder, and wear gobs of lip balm. I'd not want anyone to make eye contact with me, because it seemed as soon as they'd walk by me and look into my eyes, their eyes would then dart to my mouth corners!

Even more frustrating is when the steroid creams and the anti-fungals fail to work. I was tired of living with Angular Cheilitis and so as I sat and stared at my collection of accumulated creams to help with my condition, my mind just kept going back to what that conference lady suggested.

What stuck in my mind other than the unusual and simple nature of it was this: how could her simple solution work, when so many steroid creams and anti-fungals failed to?

I finally decided to ask a friend who worked in a medical office. I was embarrassed to ask and I could feel myself blushing as I mentioned the cure that the lady had so seriously offered me. I wanted to ask my doctor but honestly, I was afraid that they would laugh at me.

My friend contacted me the next week and she said, "Hey Heather, I looked into Angular Cheilitis and it's causes, I read over your email about the so-called cure that woman gave you, and it seems that [this nearly floored me] it may work. I see no reason why you shouldn't give it a try. It's not like it costs an arm and a leg to do it."

How could this work when all of the doctor-prescribed products failed?

In the next section, we will be going into what

causes Angular Cheilitis. Once you start to understand that, then I will go into the cure and you will see for yourself why this can work for you like it has for me.

I know that it is hard to think outside the box to try a treatment that sounds unconventional, especially when you have been working with a doctor. Let me ask you this though, how long have you been cycling through a seemingly endless collection of topical creams to cure your Angular Cheilitis to only find limited success? Are you tired of spending money on creams that just do not work?

I had a drawer filled with creams, both anti-fungal cream and steroid creams and still, I continued to have this awful problem.

4 What Causes Angular Cheilitis?

You know you have it, but why do you have it? What causes this painful and very persistent problem to manifest in the beginning?

Actually, there is no single cause; in fact, there are many factors that contribute to your Angular Cheilitis and by learning about them, you can educate yourself and take steps, all of which will make the treatment that much more effective.

Vitamin & Iron Deficiency

In order for our body to run like it should and be healthy, it needs to have a variety of vitamins and minerals. When there is a deficiency, it affects our health and wellbeing. A deficiency in both Vitamin B and in iron can contribute to Angular Cheilitis.

If you are existing on a diet of fast food and processed foods, you are very likely going to be deficient in some vital nutrients, including iron and Vitamin B. To help ensure that you are not low on either of these, take a daily vitamin that contains both iron and Vitamin B. Eating a balanced diet and taking daily vitamins will help you ensure that your body is getting the essential building blocks to health that it needs to work properly and to keep you healthy.

Skipping meals, eating too much refined sugar, eating too much processed food items such as junk food and fast food, and just generally not eating well can and will contribute to Angular Cheilitis. Make sure that you have a variety of fresh fruits and vegetables in your diet, as well as lean proteins.

Dental Problems

As we age, our bodies change and this includes our mouth. Dentures that no longer fit well can contribute to Angular Cheilitis. When dentures do not fit right, it can cause the skin around the mouth to become loose, and it will fold over around the corners of the mouth. This makes conditions perfect for bacteria to start to grow, and this can contribute to Angular Cheilitis.

Losing teeth can also change how your mouth is 'shaped', and the same problem of having loose skin around the corners of the mouth can happen. If you have lost a tooth, consider getting an implant to avoid having this type of problem manifest and if you have dentures and Angular Cheilitis, go and have them checked to see if they are still fitting properly.

Candidiasis

Candida is yeast, naturally occurring in our gastrointestinal tract. We need it to help us digest food and break down sugars. However, Candida should exist in balanced numbers, and when there are too many hanging around, it goes from a helpful, natural yeast into a fungus that can disrupt our health, known as candidiasis.

It does not take much to throw our body's balance off, causing candidiasis. A weak immune system, when our body's pH levels become too acidic, diabetes, stress and extended use of antibiotics can all cause candidiasis. Vitamin D can help a weakened immune system. I suggest doing research on this vitamin ASAP, and asking your doctor about it.

Unlike the healthy, normal yeast, Candidiasis will penetrate the wall of our digestive tract, entering our bodies. If your Angular Cheilitis is partially caused by Candidiasis, you will very often have a white tongue; a trip to the doctor to fix the underlying condition is warranted.

Cosmetics

I already mentioned how chapstick and lipstick can help spread Angular Cheilitis from one side of the mouth to the other but *any* cosmetic that goes on your lips can not only do that—if you are using old, expired lip-gloss and lipstick, that can also contribute to causing Angular Cheilitis. **Check all your makeup dates ladies, I'm just saying…**

Most of us just use our lipstick until it is gone, never paying any attention to how old it really is. I had a drawer full of half-used lipsticks because I never know what each day will bring and I like the idea of having a variety of shades from which to choose. Some of them were many years old.

I never knew that I should have been routinely throwing away old lipstick and lip-gloss instead of keeping it around! Toss your old lipsticks and lip-glosses away: only keep on hand the colors you like the best. Keeping your cosmetics long after they have passed their prime is a good way to help bacteria get a foothold in your mouth.

Parasites and Bacteria

Although our body is full of naturally occurring and helpful bacteria, it is easy for bacteria that are harmful to enter our body. Bacteria, viruses and parasites are harmful and can cause a variety of health problems, the symptoms of which will vary depending upon the type of infection.

The cure that is presented in this book can help you [yes, you!] but if the Angular Cheilitis comes back and keeps recurring, then there could be a medical reason for it. Bacteria and parasites are a possibility for some Angular Cheilitis sufferers.

Easy way to remove parasites? Eat lots of raw vegetables—I personally eat coleslaw every week, but if you don't like it, you may want to try sauerkraut, vinegary olives or other vinegary things.

What are some of the symptoms to look out for, in addition to Angular Cheilitis?

- Stomach cramps
- Gas
- Anemia
- Skin problems or allergies
- Loss of appetite or sudden change in appetite
- Arthritis
- Bloating
- Mouth blisters
- Trouble concentrating
- Constipation
- Diarrhea
- Fatigue
- Digestion troubles
- Headaches
- IBS (Irritable Bowel)
- Nausea
- Skin rashes
- Insomnia
- Weight loss (sudden and unexplained)
- Muscle pain
- Loss of memory

If you find that you have more than one of the above symptoms and that they all started around the same time, seek medical attention to rule out a bacterial infection or parasites.

In the meantime, two natural remedies for parasites and harmful bacteria are licorice root and cloves.

By chewing one clove every day, you can help rid yourself of harmful intestinal bacteria. Clove is also a natural pain reliever. Licorice root can help lower inflammation, and act as an anti-viral agent and helps to heal stomach ulcers. *It should not be taken by anybody who has a problem with water retention or anybody with high blood pressure.*

How I Finally Got Rid Of Angular Cheilitis Once and For All!

HEATHER KALE

5 Curing your Angular Cheilitis

Now that you understand some of the things and conditions that can cause or contribute to having Angular Cheilitis, it is time to go into the cure. If you are like me, and have tried every recommended product with no results, you are probably feeling skeptical. Your skepticism will only increase when I tell you what the actual cure is but remember that I had the very same reaction.

I remember thinking, "That will never work", "What an odd solution", and "I'll never try that." Then, out of frustration, I did try it. Not only did my mouth start to feel better within a day, but also it started to look better. No more pain when I opened my mouth, no deep splits that showed when I talked. I no longer felt self-conscious every time I was out in public.

Before you roll your eyes at what I have to say, just try it! That is all I ask, just try it and see for yourself because honestly, I can extol the virtues of this cure until I am blue in the face but hearing about something is not the same as trying it for yourself.

Try it, and you will soon be telling everybody that

you know about the simple and unusual cure that finally ended your Angular Cheilitis problem.

What you will need

This subchapter is all about what you will need in order to use this cure. Chances are that you have most of these things around the house already and if not, none of the necessary items is very expensive. When I promised you a simple cure that is just what I meant.

- **Plain Tissues**

You will need to have plain tissues, without lotion or fragrances. Using the kind with lotion or with scents will only hinder the cure, not help it. All you need is a box of plain, every day tissues.

- **Two bowls and a nailbrush**

You will need two everyday bowls that have been washed and sterilized. You need to make sure that they are free of dust or anything else that can contaminate them, so instead of just reaching for two bowls from the cabinet, you need to sterilize them right before using this cure. Take each bowl, wash it with a little liquid dishwashing soap and then use boiling water to rinse out the bowls. The best way to do this is to wash the bowls, then set them in the dish drainer or sink, and *then*

pour the boiling water over them.
Do not attempt to hold the bowls and then pour boiling water into them; you can easily burn yourself that way. Please use a new nailbrush!

• **Plate**

You will need a medium to small sized plate, such as a coffee cup saucer or a small sandwich plate. Wash and sterilize the plate before using just as instructed to do with the two bowls above.

• **Liquid dishwashing soap**

This is the part where I originally shook my head because never would I have thought that somebody would recommend using liquid dishwashing soap instead of regular hand soap. Hand soap is for hands, this is for dishes but yet, it is very effective and yes, I was surprised as well! Dishwashing soap has everything needed to help clean and kill germs, making it perfectly suited to this cure. The brand does not necessarily matter; you just need to have a bottle on hand for this to work. I have spoken to people who tried the cure using soap or antibacterial soap instead of the liquid dishwashing soap and they **did not get the same results**. Bottom line is that the liquid dishwashing soap works far better than hand soap for this cure.

- **Antibacterial mouthwash**

You will need to not only have clean hands, but a clean mouth prior to starting this treatment. This ensures that a significant portion of the bacteria that is in your mouth will be killed prior to beginning each treatment.

- **Petroleum Jelly**

You can use Vaseline or any other brand as long as it is white petroleum jelly. One of the problems with petroleum jelly is that to use it, you usually just stick a finger in the jar and take out how much you need. *If your finger is dirty, you have contaminated the container.* Because bacteria are a big part of the root problem of Angular Cheilitis, my recommendation is that you get a **brand new jar of petroleum jelly** just for this cure. This way, you know that you are not using older petroleum jelly that may or may not already contain dirt and germs. This is a vital part of the cure. The bacteria that are responsible for Angular Cheilitis are fungal bacteria and they need a moist environment in which to live, thrive and multiply. If you take away that environment, they will die and that is what the petroleum jelly is for.

When applied, it will create a waterproof layer, sealing off the bacteria from the moisture that they need to live. Remove the moisture, and you get rid of the bacteria that cause AC.

Curing your Angular Cheilitis

You may be wondering, after reading the list of what you need to cure your Angular Cheilitis how any of those will come together to cure this painful and unsightly condition.

I know, I was wondering that myself! Everything on that list is very specifically designed towards being **clean and hygienic**.

You will need a few hours at home to do this. You can do it on a weekend morning, or at home after work but you will need about three hours to apply and leave the treatment in order to see results. Make sure that you have done all of your errands and have a chunk of time to let the process work once applied. You can certainly do things around the house once you have applied the treatment, but because you will be applying the treatment to your mouth and lips, you will not want to be out running around.

When you use the cure, **before you even sterilize the plate and the bowls, you need to have a clean, germ free work environment.** You can use your bathroom counter, that is where I preferred to use the remedy, or you can use your kitchen. **You need to be in close proximity to a clean sink**, which is why these two rooms are recommended. **Please have**

clean cotton towels handy as well.
Make sure that you have cleaned the area well, using a counter cleaner that is designed to kill germs and bacteria. A clean work surface is necessary. You are trying to rid the area of bacteria, so always clean the sink and the counter before beginning.

Once you have the counter and sink cleaned, wash your hands with hot water and the liquid dishwashing soap. Use a clean nailbrush to really clean under and around your nails. Even if you have short nails, dead skin cells and dirt will accumulate there, a breeding ground for germs and more bacteria.

Once your hands are cleaned, you can wash and sterilize the bowls and plates and then place them on the counter; they should be placed near each other.

Keep the nailbrush and the liquid dishwashing soap [and clean cotton towels!] handy because this cure is in steps and *in between each step, you will need to wash your hands and scrub your nails.* This prevents you from transferring any bacteria that could be on your hands onto your mouth.

Now, you also need to have a clean mouth. Start off by brushing your teeth and then also brush your tongue. After brushing, floss your teeth and then brush your teeth again. Swish your mouth out using the mouthwash next, making sure to swish for at least thirty seconds.

Now, clean your hands again. I know that a lot of these steps might be repetitive and on the surface, seem redundant but they are not. It is easy to pick up new bacteria and germs on your hands and you do not want that in your mouth, it will only work against you or make the cure ineffective. It is set up this way for a reason; it works, but only if you follow it exactly. If you try to cut corners and skip some of the hand washings, it can hinder the healing of your Angular Cheilitis.

Squeeze some of the liquid dishwashing soap onto the plate. You do not need to fill the plate, just squeeze out a small amount, like a teaspoon or so. There is no exact measurement but you do not want to waste the soap, so just about 'a teaspoon' is a good amount.

Wash your hands again with the liquid dish soap, scrubbing around and under your nails. You can now fill the bowls with hot water. The water needs to be hot, but not so hot that you will burn yourself when you touch it. The idea is to have the water as hot as you can stand it without burning yourself.

Once again, wash your hands paying careful attention to your nails but do not dry your hands after.

Using the first bowl only, dip your fingers into

the bowl and wet your lips, making sure that the corners of your mouth get plenty of water. Once again, only use the first bowl; it is important that you do not use both bowls at this stage, just the first one.

The hot water does two things. First, it helps to wash away bacteria around the mouth and on the lips; this is why the water needs to be hot. Secondly, the hot water is necessary to soften the skin of your lips and your mouth, especially in the corners. That is why you need to really make sure that you dampen the corners of your mouth, especially if you have sores or cuts from the Angular Cheilitis.

The next step is where many people just shake their head and look at me as if I am crazy. It sounds crazy but it works. Only because I was so desperate for a solution did I finally decide to try this crazy-sounding cure and it worked so as crazy as it sounds, I really hope you do give it a try!

Dip your finger into the liquid dish soap that you have on the small plate and then, with your mouth closed, rub the liquid dish soap into the corners of your mouth, making sure to work it into any sores that you have. It is okay to dip your finger back into the plate to get more.

Keep your mouth tightly closed as you rub the liquid dish soap into each corner of your mouth.

You need to massage the dish soap into each corner for about a minute. If you get soap inside your mouth (yuk!), just rinse your mouth out until you have gotten rid of the soap and then *start over from step one, with freshly sterilized bowls and a freshly sterilized plate.*

The soap will sting so expect it to hurt some. This is normal. You are putting soap in open sores but it will help kill the bacteria that are causing the sores so it is necessary.

Wash your hands again, including scrubbing your nails--but do not dry them!

Use the clean, hot water from the second bowl to wash away all of the liquid dish soap off of your face. You need to make sure that all of the soap is gone, so really rinse your mouth and the corners of your mouth well with the water from the second bowl by splashing water onto your mouth and lips.

Wash your hands again, including your nails and then dry your hands using a clean dry towel. Use a new towel each treatment, you need to ensure it is a fresh, clean towel.

Use the plain tissues and begin to dry your lips and the corners of your mouth. Do not wipe the tissues across your mouth because this spreads bacteria. Take a clean tissue, dab at your lower lip, in the center, and then work your way into one corner of your mouth. Dab at your mouth, then get a new tissue; you do not want to use the same tissue to dab at more than one area of your mouth.

When you get to the corner of your mouth, repeat the process to dry off the rest of your lower lip and then repeat for your top lip. You will go through many tissues for this step and that is okay. It is better to use many tissues than to spread the bacteria and make your Angular Cheilitis worse. Really make sure that the corners of your mouth are dry.

Once again, wash your hands, scrub your nails and then dry your hands.

Dip a finger into the petroleum jelly and then apply it to your lips, your chin, under your nose and most importantly, to the sores and cuts from the Angular Cheilitis. You need to have a thick layer on, so do not skimp on how much you use.

Take a selfie now and post it online [seriously I am kidding!]. **You need to leave the petroleum jelly on for around three hours.**

After three hours, you can begin to prepare for the second part of the treatment.

Clean the counter and sink just as you did before and wash and sterilize the two bowls and the plate.

Set the two bowls on the counter and fill with hot water, but not so hot that it will burn you; and then squeeze a small amount of the dish soap onto the plate.

Just like you did for step one, wash your hands with liquid dish soap, scrub your nails, and then dry them on a new, clean towel.

Use tissues to remove as much petroleum jelly as you can, being gentle as you carefully wipe it off.

Wash your hands but do not dry them; and then use the water from the first bowl to wash your mouth and lips.

Once again, wash your hands and scrub your nails but do not dry your hands. Use the liquid dish soap from the plate and rub it into your lips and corners of your mouth while keeping your mouth tightly closed to prevent the soap from getting into your mouth.

Wash your hands and scrub your nails and then use the water from the second bowl to wash away all of the soap.

Do not touch your mouth for the next half hour and do not blot or dab with tissues but instead, **let it air dry.** This will take about half an hour.

Within 24 hours, you should start to notice a reduction in redness and inflammation, and your sores should appear much less noticeable.

If you have Angular Cheilitis that is severe and this cure does not fully work, then do the entire process again, but instead of leaving the petroleum jelly on for three hours, leave it on overnight. Make sure that you place a thick towel over your pillow to prevent the petroleum jelly from getting on your pillow.

I recommend doing this treatment at least once a day, twice if you have the time; but if you have severe AC, I recommend you do this for about two weeks. You should see a vast improvement. If you are not fully healed after three weeks, then continue to do this daily and be sure to include several overnight treatments as well.

In my humble opinion, this method should work for most Angular Cheilitis sufferers.

How I Finally Got Rid Of Angular Cheilitis Once and For All!

HEATHER KALE

6 Conclusion

This is the method that I used to cure my Angular Cheilitis and it worked.

I saw and felt an improvement by the next morning! After three weeks, my Angular Cheilitis was nearly gone. Now mind you, I did have a *severe* case and I had to do several overnight treatments so I'd wait for the weekend to do this. I performed the treatment morning and night, and that really helped me cure the last of it.

Keep in mind that your Angular Cheilitis could be lingering due to some of the underlying reasons that I listed in a prior chapter-**please go over those and share them with others.** Unless you address those issues, it will return and you will need to use the treatment again.

Good luck to you and I wish you the best Health, Wealth and Happiness.

THE END

www.ingramcontent.com/pod-product-compliance
Lightning Source LLC
Chambersburg PA
CBHW070504290526
45790CB00003B/1097